INDIAN COOKBOOK

2021

FLAVORFUL INDIAN RECIPES

SECOND EDITION

JANE PETERSON

Table of Contents

No-Oil Chicken 12

    Ingredients 12

    Method 12

Kozi Varatha Curry 13

    Ingredients 13

    Method 14

Chicken Stew 15

    Ingredients 15

    Method 16

Chicken Himani 17

    Ingredients 17

    For the marinade: 17

    Method 17

White Chicken 18

    Ingredients 18

    Method 19

Chicken in Red Masala 20

    Ingredients 20

    Method 21

Chicken Jhalfrezie 22

    Ingredients 22

    Method 23

Simple Chicken Curry 24

Ingredients 24

Method.. 25

Sour Chicken Curry.. 26

Ingredients 26

Method.. 27

Anjeer Dry Chicken.. 28

Ingredients 28

For the marinade: 28

Method.. 29

Chicken Yoghurt 30

Ingredients 30

Method.. 31

Spicy Fried Chicken 32

Ingredients 32

Method.. 33

Chicken Supreme 34

Ingredients 34

Method.. 35

Chicken Vindaloo 36

Ingredients 36

Method.. 37

Caramelized Chicken 38

Ingredients 38

Method.. 39

Cashew Chicken 40

Ingredients 40

Method.. 41

Quick Chicken 42

    Ingredients 42

    Method 43

Coorgi Chicken Curry 44

    Ingredients 44

    Method 45

Pan Chicken 46

    Ingredients 46

    Method 47

Spinach Chicken 48

    Ingredients 48

    Method 49

Chicken Indienne 50

    Ingredients 50

    For the spice mixture: 50

    Method 51

Kori Gassi 52

    Ingredients 52

    Method 53

Chicken Ghezado 54

    Ingredients 54

    Method 54

Chicken in Tomato Gravy 55

    Ingredients 55

    Method 56

Shahenshah Murgh 57

    Ingredients 57

Method..58

Chicken do Pyaaza...59

    Ingredients 59

    Method..60

Bengali Chicken 61

    Ingredients 61

    Method..61

Lasooni Murgh 62

    Ingredients 62

    Method..63

Chicken Cafreal 64

    Ingredients 64

    For the marinade: 64

    Method..65

Chicken with Apricots 66

    Ingredients 66

    Method..67

Grilled Chicken 68

    Ingredients 68

    Method..69

Pepper Duck Roast 70

    Ingredients 70

    Method..71

Bhuna Chicken...72

    Ingredients 72

    Method..73

Chicken Curry with Eggs...74

Ingredients..74

Method 75

Chicken Fried with Spices 76

Ingredients..76

For the marinade: 76

Method 77

Goan Kombdi 78

Ingredients..78

Method 79

South Chicken Curry 80

Ingredients..80

Method 81

Nizami Chicken 82

Ingredients..82

For the spice mixture: 82

Method 83

Duck Buffad 84

Ingredients..84

Method 85

Adraki Murgh..86

Ingredients..86

Method 86

Bharva Murgh 87

Ingredients..87

Method 88

Malaidar Murgh 89

Ingredients..89

Method 90

Bombay Chicken Curry 91

    Ingredients 91

    Method 92

Durbari Chicken 93

    Ingredients 93

    Method 94

Duck Fry 95

    Ingredients 95

    Method 95

Coriander Garlic Chicken 96

    Ingredients 96

    Method 97

Masala Duck 98

    Ingredients 98

    Method 99

Mustard Chicken 100

    Ingredients 100

    Method 101

Murgh Lassanwallah 102

    Ingredients 102

    Method 103

Pepper Chicken Chettinad 104

    Ingredients 104

    Method 105

Chicken Mince with Eggs 106

    Ingredients 106

Method 107

Dry Chicken 108

Ingredients 108

For the marinade: 108

Method 109

Prawn Curry Rosachi 110

Ingredients 110

Method 111

Fish Stuffed with Dates & Almonds 112

Ingredients 112

Method 112

Tandoori Fish 114

Ingredients 114

Method 114

Fish with Vegetables 115

Ingredients 115

Method 116

Tandoor Gulnar 117

Ingredients 117

For the first marinade: 117

For the second marinade: 117

Prawns in Green Masala 118

Ingredients 118

Method 119

Fish Cutlet 120

Ingredients 120

Method 121

Parsi Fish Sas 122

    Ingredients 122

    Method.. 123

Peshawari Machhi... 124

    Ingredients 124

    Method.. 124

Crab Curry 125

    Ingredients 125

    Method.. 126

Mustard Fish 127

    Ingredients 127

    Method.. 127

Meen Vattichathu 128

    Ingredients 128

    Method.. 129

No-Oil Chicken

Serves 4

Ingredients

400g/14oz yoghurt

1 tsp chilli powder

1 tsp ginger paste

1 tsp garlic paste

2 green chillies, finely chopped

50g/1¾oz coriander leaves, ground

1 tsp garam masala

Salt to taste

750g/1lb 10oz boneless chicken, chopped into 8 pieces

Method

- Mix together all the ingredients, except the chicken. Marinate the chicken with this mixture overnight.

- Cook the marinated chicken in a saucepan on a medium heat for 40 minutes, stirring frequently. Serve hot.

Kozi Varatha Curry

(Kairali Chicken Curry from Kerala)

Serves 4

Ingredients

60ml/2fl oz refined vegetable oil

7.5cm/3in root ginger, finely chopped

15 garlic cloves, finely chopped

8 shallots, sliced

3 green chillies, slit lengthways

1kg/2¼lb chicken, chopped into 12 pieces

¾ tsp turmeric

Salt to taste

2 tbsp ground coriander

1 tbsp garam masala

½ tsp cumin seeds

750ml/1¼ pints coconut milk

5-6 curry leaves

Method

- Heat the oil in a saucepan. Add the ginger and garlic. Fry on a medium heat for 30 seconds.

- Add the shallots and green chillies. Stir-fry for a minute.

- Add the chicken, turmeric, salt, ground coriander, garam masala and cumin seeds. Mix well. Cover with a lid and cook on a low heat for 20 minutes. Add the coconut milk. Simmer for 20 minutes.

- Garnish with the curry leaves and serve hot.

Chicken Stew

Ingredients

1 tbsp refined vegetable oil

2 cloves

2.5cm/1in cinnamon

6 black peppercorns

3 bay leaves

2 large onions, chopped into 8 pieces

1 tsp ginger paste

1 tsp garlic paste

8 chicken drumsticks

200g/7oz frozen mixed vegetables

250ml/8fl oz water

Salt to taste

2 tsp plain white flour, dissolved in 360ml/12fl oz milk

Method

- Heat the oil in a saucepan. Add the cloves, cinnamon, peppercorns and bay leaves. Let them splutter for 30 seconds.

- Add the onions, ginger paste and garlic paste. Fry for 2 minutes.

- Add the remaining ingredients, except the flour mixture. Cover with a lid and simmer for 30 minutes. Add the flour mixture. Mix well.

- Simmer for 10 minutes, stirring frequently. Serve hot.

Chicken Himani

(Cardamom Chicken)

Serves 4

Ingredients

1kg/2¼lb chicken, chopped into 10 pieces

3 tbsp refined vegetable oil

¼ tsp ground green cardamom

Salt to taste

For the marinade:

1 tsp ginger paste

1 tsp garlic paste

200g/7oz yoghurt

2 tbsp mint leaves, ground

Method

- Mix all the marinade ingredients together. Marinate the chicken with this mixture for 4 hours.

- Heat the oil in a saucepan. Add the marinated chicken and fry on a low heat for 10 minutes. Add the cardamom and salt. Mix well and cook for 30 minutes, stirring frequently. Serve hot.

17

White Chicken

Ingredients

750g/1lb 10oz boneless chicken, chopped

1 tsp ginger paste

1 tsp garlic paste

1 tbsp ghee

2 cloves

2.5cm/1in cinnamon

8 black peppercorns

2 bay leaves

Salt to taste

250ml/8fl oz water

30g/1oz cashew nuts, ground

10-12 almonds, ground

1 tbsp single cream

Method

- Marinate the chicken with the ginger paste and garlic paste for 30 minutes.

- Heat the ghee in a saucepan. Add the cloves, cinnamon, peppercorns, bay leaves and salt. Let them splutter for 15 seconds.

- Add the marinated chicken and water. Simmer for 30 minutes. Add the cashew nuts, almonds and cream. Cook for 5 minutes and serve hot.

Chicken in Red Masala

Serves 4

Ingredients

3 tbsp refined vegetable oil

2 large onions, finely sliced

1 tbsp poppy seeds

5 dry red chillies

50g/1¾oz fresh coconut, grated

2.5cm/1in cinnamon

2 tsp tamarind paste

6 garlic cloves

500g/1lb 2oz chicken, chopped

2 tomatoes, finely sliced

1 tbsp ground coriander

1 tsp ground cumin

500ml/16fl oz water

Salt to taste

Method

- Heat the oil in a saucepan. Fry the onions on a medium heat till brown. Add the poppy seeds, chillies, coconut and cinnamon. Fry for 3 minutes.

- Add the tamarind paste and garlic. Mix well and grind into a paste.

- Mix this paste with all the remaining ingredients. Cook the mixture in a saucepan on a low heat for 40 minutes. Serve hot.

Chicken Jhalfrezie

(Chicken in Thick Tomato Gravy)

Serves 4

Ingredients

3 tbsp refined vegetable oil

3 large onions, finely chopped

2.5cm/1in root ginger, finely sliced

1 tsp garlic paste

1kg/2¼lb chicken, chopped into 8 pieces

½ tsp turmeric

3 tsp ground coriander

1 tsp ground cumin

4 tomatoes, blanched and puréed

Salt to taste

Method

- Heat the oil in a saucepan. Add the onions, ginger and garlic paste. Fry on a medium heat till the onions are brown.

- Add the chicken, turmeric, ground coriander and ground cumin. Fry for 5 minutes.

- Add the tomato purée and salt. Mix well and cook on a low heat for 40 minutes, stirring occasionally. Serve hot.

Simple Chicken Curry

Serves 4

Ingredients

2 tbsp refined vegetable oil

2 large onions, sliced

½ tsp turmeric

1 tsp ginger paste

1 tsp garlic paste

6 green chillies, sliced

750g/1lb 10oz chicken, chopped into 8 pieces

125g/4½oz yoghurt

125g/4½oz khoya*

Salt to taste

50g/1¾oz coriander leaves, finely chopped

Method

- Heat the oil in a saucepan. Add the onions. Fry till they turn translucent.

- Add the turmeric, ginger paste, garlic paste and green chillies. Fry on a medium heat for 2 minutes. Add the chicken and fry for 5 minutes.

- Add the yoghurt, khoya and salt. Mix thoroughly. Cover with a lid and cook on a low heat for 30 minutes, stirring occasionally.

- Garnish with the coriander leaves. Serve hot.

Sour Chicken Curry

Serves 4

Ingredients

1kg/2¼lb chicken, chopped into 8 pieces

Salt to taste

½ tsp turmeric

4 tbsp refined vegetable oil

3 onions, finely chopped

8 curry leaves

3 tomatoes, finely chopped

1 tsp ginger paste

1 tsp garlic paste

1 tbsp ground coriander

1 tsp garam masala

1 tbsp tamarind paste

½ tbsp ground black pepper

250ml/8fl oz water

Method

- Marinate the chicken pieces with the salt and turmeric for 30 minutes.

- Heat the oil in a saucepan. Add the onions and curry leaves. Fry on a low heat till the onions are translucent.

- Add all the remaining ingredients and the marinated chicken. Mix well, cover with a lid and simmer for 40 minutes. Serve hot.

Anjeer Dry Chicken

(Dry Chicken with Figs)

Serves 4

Ingredients

750g/1lb 10oz chicken, chopped into 12 pieces

4 tbsp ghee

2 large onions, finely chopped

250ml/8fl oz water

Salt to taste

For the marinade:

10 dry figs, soaked for 1 hour

1 tsp ginger paste

1 tsp garlic paste

200g/7oz yoghurt

1½ tsp garam masala

2 tbsp single cream

Method

- Mix all the marinade ingredients together. Marinate the chicken with this mixture for an hour.

- Heat the ghee in a saucepan. Fry the onions on a medium heat till brown.

- Add the marinated chicken, water and salt. Mix well, cover with a lid and simmer for 40 minutes. Serve hot.

Chicken Yoghurt

Serves 4

Ingredients

30g/1oz mint leaves, finely chopped

30g/1oz coriander leaves, chopped

2 tsp ginger paste

2 tsp garlic paste

400g/14oz yoghurt

200g/7oz tomato purée

Juice of 1 lemon

1kg/2¼lb chicken, chopped into 12 pieces

2 tbsp refined vegetable oil

4 large onions, finely chopped

Salt to taste

Method

- Grind the mint leaves and coriander leaves to a fine paste. Mix this with the ginger paste, garlic paste, yoghurt, tomato purée and lemon juice. Marinate the chicken with this mixture for 3 hours.

- Heat the oil in a saucepan. Fry the onions on a medium heat till brown.

- Add the marinated chicken. Cover with a lid and simmer for 40 minutes, stirring occasionally. Serve hot.

Spicy Fried Chicken

Serves 4

Ingredients

1 tsp ginger paste

2 tsp garlic paste

2 green chillies, finely chopped

1 tsp chilli powder

1 tsp garam masala

2 tsp lemon juice

½ tsp turmeric

Salt to taste

1kg/2¼lb chicken, chopped into 8 pieces

Refined vegetable oil for deep-frying

Breadcrumbs, to coat

Method

- Mix the ginger paste, garlic paste, green chillies, chilli powder, garam masala, lemon juice, turmeric and salt together. Marinate the chicken with this mixture for 3 hours.

- Heat the oil in a frying pan. Coat each marinated chicken piece with the breadcrumbs and deep fry on a medium heat till golden brown.

- Drain on absorbent paper and serve hot.

Chicken Supreme

Serves 4

Ingredients

1 tsp ginger paste

1 tsp garlic paste

1kg/2¼lb chicken, chopped into 8 pieces

200g/7oz yoghurt

Salt to taste

250ml/8fl oz water

2 tbsp refined vegetable oil

2 large onions, sliced

4 red chillies

5cm/2in cinnamon

2 black cardamom pods

4 cloves

1 tbsp chana dhal*, dry roasted

Method

- Mix the ginger paste and garlic paste together. Marinate the chicken with this mixture for 30 minutes. Add the yoghurt, salt and water. Set aside.

- Heat the oil in a saucepan. Add the onions, chillies, cinnamon, cardamom, cloves and chana dhal. Fry for 3-4 minutes on a low heat.

- Grind to a paste and add to the chicken mixture. Mix well.

- Cook on a low heat for 30 minutes. Serve hot.

Chicken Vindaloo

(Spicy Goan-style Chicken Curry)

Serves 4

Ingredients

60ml/2fl oz malt vinegar

1 tbsp cumin seeds

1 tsp peppercorns

6 red chillies

1 tsp turmeric

Salt to taste

4 tbsp refined vegetable oil

3 large onions, finely chopped

1kg/2¼lb chicken, chopped into 8 pieces

Method

- Grind the vinegar with the cumin seeds, peppercorns, chillies, turmeric and salt to a smooth paste. Set aside.

- Heat the oil in a saucepan. Add the onions and fry till translucent. Add the vinegar-cumin seeds paste. Mix well and fry for 4-5 minutes.

- Add the chicken and cook on a low heat for 30 minutes. Serve hot.

Caramelized Chicken

Serves 4

Ingredients

200g/7oz yoghurt

1 tsp ginger paste

1 tsp garlic paste

2 tbsp ground coriander

1 tsp ground cumin

1½ tsp garam masala

Salt to taste

1kg/2¼lb chicken, chopped into 8 pieces

3 tbsp refined vegetable oil

2 tsp sugar

3 cloves

2.5cm/1in cinnamon

6 black peppercorns

Method

- Mix together the yoghurt, ginger paste, garlic paste, ground coriander, ground cumin, garam masala and salt. Marinate the chicken with this mixture overnight.

- Heat the oil in a saucepan. Add the sugar, cloves, cinnamon and peppercorns. Fry for a minute. Add the marinated chicken and cook on a low heat for 40 minutes. Serve hot.

Cashew Chicken

Serves 4

Ingredients

1kg/2¼lb chicken, chopped into 12 pieces

Salt to taste

1 tsp ginger paste

1 tsp garlic paste

4 tbsp refined vegetable oil

4 large onions, sliced

15 cashew nuts, ground to a paste

6 red chillies, soaked for 15 minutes

2 tsp ground cumin

60ml/2fl oz ketchup

500ml/16fl oz water

Method

- Marinate the chicken with the salt and ginger and garlic pastes for 1 hour.

- Heat the oil in a saucepan. Fry the onions on a medium heat till brown.

- Add the cashew nuts, chillies, cumin and ketchup. Cook for 5 minutes.

- Add the chicken and the water. Simmer for 40 minutes and serve hot.

Quick Chicken

Serves 4

Ingredients

4 tbsp refined vegetable oil

6 red chillies

6 black peppercorns

1 tsp coriander seeds

1 tsp cumin seeds

2.5cm/1in cinnamon

4 cloves

1 tsp turmeric

8 garlic cloves

1 tsp tamarind paste

4 medium-sized onions, finely sliced

2 large tomatoes, finely chopped

1kg/2¼lb chicken, chopped into 12 pieces

250ml/8fl oz water

Salt to taste

Method

- Heat half a tbsp of oil in a saucepan. Add the red chillies, peppercorns, coriander seeds, cumin seeds, cinnamon and cloves. Fry them on a medium heat for 2-3 minutes.
- Add the turmeric, garlic and tamarind paste. Grind the mixture to a smooth paste. Set aside.
- Heat the remaining oil in a saucepan. Add the onions and fry them on a medium heat till they are brown. Add the tomatoes and sauté for 3-4 minutes.
- Add the chicken and sauté for 4-5 minutes.
- Add the water and salt. Mix well and cover with a lid. Simmer for 40 minutes, stirring occasionally.
- Serve hot.

Coorgi Chicken Curry

Serves 4

Ingredients

1kg/2¼lb chicken, chopped into 12 pieces

Salt to taste

1 tsp turmeric

50g/1¾oz grated coconut

3 tbsp refined vegetable oil

1 tsp garlic paste

2 large onions, finely sliced

1 tsp ground cumin

1 tsp ground coriander

360ml/12fl oz water

Method

- Marinate the chicken with the salt and turmeric for an hour. Set aside.

- Grind the coconut with enough water to form a smooth paste.

- Heat the oil in a saucepan. Add the coconut paste with the garlic paste, onions, ground cumin and coriander. Fry on a low heat for 4-5 minutes.

- Add the marinated chicken. Mix well and fry for 4-5 minutes. Add the water, cover with a lid and simmer for 40 minutes. Serve hot.

Pan Chicken

Serves 4

Ingredients

4 tbsp refined vegetable oil

1 tsp ginger paste

1 tsp garlic paste

2 large onions, finely chopped

1 tsp garam masala

1½ tbsp cashew nuts, ground

1½ tbsp melon seeds*, ground

1 tsp ground coriander

500g/1lb 2oz boneless chicken

200g/7oz tomato purée

2 chicken stock cubes

250ml/8fl oz water

Salt to taste

Method

- Heat the oil in a saucepan. Add the ginger paste, garlic paste, onions and garam masala. Fry for 2-3 minutes on a low heat. Add the cashew nuts, melon seeds and ground coriander. Fry for 2 minutes.
- Add the chicken and fry for 5 minutes. Add the tomato purée, stock cubes, water and salt. Cover and simmer for 40 minutes. Serve hot.

Spinach Chicken

Serves 4

Ingredients

3 tbsp refined vegetable oil

6 cloves

5cm/2in cinnamon

2 bay leaves

2 large onions, finely chopped

12 garlic cloves, finely chopped

400g/14oz spinach, coarsely chopped

200g/7oz yoghurt

250ml/8fl oz water

750g/1lb 10oz chicken, chopped into 8 pieces

Salt to taste

Method

- Heat 2 tbsp oil in a saucepan. Add the cloves, cinnamon and bay leaves. Let them splutter for 15 seconds.
- Add the onions and fry them on a medium heat till they turn translucent.
- Add the garlic and spinach. Mix well. Cook for 5-6 minutes. Cool and grind with enough water to make a smooth paste.
- Heat the remaining oil in a saucepan. Add the spinach paste and fry for 3-4 minutes. Add the yoghurt and water. Cook for 5-6 minutes. Add the chicken and salt. Cook on a low heat for 40 minutes. Serve hot.

Chicken Indienne

Serves 4

Ingredients

4-5 tbsp refined vegetable oil

4 large onions, minced

1kg/2¼lb chicken, chopped into 10 pieces

Salt to taste

500ml/16fl oz water

For the spice mixture:

2.5cm/1in root ginger

10 garlic cloves

1 tbsp garam masala

2 tsp fennel seeds

1½ tbsp coriander seeds

60ml/2fl oz water

Method

- Grind the spice mixture ingredients into a smooth paste. Set aside.
- Heat the oil in a saucepan. Fry the onions on a medium heat till brown.
- Add the spice mixture paste, the chicken and salt. Fry for 5-6 minutes. Add the water. Cover and cook for 40 minutes. Serve hot.

Kori Gassi

(Mangalorean Chicken with Curry)

Serves 4

Ingredients

4 tbsp refined vegetable oil

6 whole red chillies

1 tsp black peppercorns

4 tsp coriander seeds

2 tsp cumin seeds

150g/5½oz fresh coconut, grated

8 garlic cloves

500ml/16fl oz water

3 large onions, finely chopped

1 tsp turmeric

1kg/2¼lb chicken, chopped into 8 pieces

2 tsp tamarind paste

Salt to taste

Method

- Heat 1 tsp oil in a saucepan. Add the red chillies, peppercorns, coriander seeds and cumin seeds. Let them splutter for 15 seconds.

- Grind this mixture to a paste with the coconut, garlic and half the water.

- Heat the remaining oil in a saucepan. Add the onions, turmeric and the coconut paste. Fry on a medium heat for 5-6 minutes.

- Add the chicken, tamarind paste, salt and the remaining water. Mix well. Cover with a lid and simmer for 40 minutes. Serve hot.

Chicken Ghezado

(Goan-style Chicken)

Serves 4

Ingredients

3 tbsp refined vegetable oil

2 large onions, finely chopped

1 tsp ginger paste

1 tsp garlic paste

2 tomatoes, finely chopped

1kg/2¼lb chicken, chopped into 8 pieces

1 tbsp ground coriander

2 tbsp garam masala

Salt to taste

250ml/8fl oz water

Method

- Heat the oil in a saucepan. Add the onions, ginger paste and garlic paste. Fry for 2 minutes. Add the tomatoes and chicken. Fry for 5 minutes.
- Add all the remaining ingredients. Simmer for 40 minutes and serve hot.

Chicken in Tomato Gravy

Serves 4

Ingredients

1 tbsp ghee

2.5cm/1in root ginger, finely chopped

10 garlic cloves, finely chopped

2 large onions, finely chopped

4 red chillies

1 tsp garam masala

1 tsp turmeric

800g/1¾lb tomato purée

1kg/2¼lb chicken, chopped into 8 pieces

Salt to taste

200g/7oz yoghurt

Method

- Heat the ghee in a saucepan. Add the ginger, garlic, onions, red chillies, garam masala and turmeric. Fry on a medium heat for 3 minutes.
- Add the tomato purée and fry for 4 minutes on a low heat.
- Add the chicken, salt and yoghurt. Mix thoroughly.
- Cover and simmer for 40 minutes, stirring occasionally. Serve hot.

Shahenshah Murgh

(Chicken cooked in Special Gravy)

Serves 4

Ingredients

250g/9oz peanuts, soaked for 4 hours

60g/2oz raisins

4 green chillies, slit lengthways

1 tbsp cumin seeds

4 tbsp ghee

1 tbsp ground cinnamon

3 large onions, finely chopped

1kg/2¼lb chicken, chopped in 12 pieces

Salt to taste

Method

- Drain the peanuts and grind them with the raisins, green chillies, cumin seeds and enough water to form a smooth paste. Set aside.
- Heat the ghee in a saucepan. Add the ground cinnamon. Let it splutter for 30 seconds.
- Add the onions and the ground peanut-raisin paste. Fry for 2-3 minutes.
- Add the chicken and salt. Mix well. Cook on a low heat for 40 minutes, stirring occasionally. Serve hot.

Chicken do Pyaaza

(Chicken with Onions)

Serves 4

Ingredients

4 tbsp ghee plus extra for deep frying

4 cloves

½ tsp fennel seeds

1 tsp ground coriander

1 tsp ground black pepper

2.5cm/1in root ginger, finely chopped

8 garlic cloves, finely chopped

4 large onions, sliced

1kg/2¼lb chicken, chopped into 12 pieces

½ tsp turmeric

4 tomatoes, finely chopped

Salt to taste

Method

- Heat 4 tbsp ghee in a saucepan. Add the cloves, fennel seeds, ground coriander and pepper. Let them splutter for 15 seconds.
- Add the ginger, garlic and onions. Fry on a medium heat for 1-2 minutes.
- Add the chicken, turmeric, tomatoes and salt. Mix well. Cook on a low heat for 30 minutes, stirring frequently. Serve hot.

Bengali Chicken

Serves 4

Ingredients

300g/10oz yoghurt

1 tsp ginger paste

1 tsp garlic paste

3 large onions, 1 grated plus 2 finely chopped

1 tsp turmeric

2 tsp chilli powder

Salt to taste

1kg/2¼lb chicken, chopped into 12 pieces

4 tbsp mustard oil

500ml/16fl oz water

Method

- Mix the yoghurt, ginger paste, garlic paste, onion, turmeric, chilli powder and salt together. Marinate the chicken with this mixture for 30 minutes.
- Heat the oil in a saucepan. Add the chopped onions and fry till brown.
- Add the marinated chicken, water and salt. Mix well. Cover with a lid and simmer for 40 minutes. Serve hot.

Lasooni Murgh

(Chicken cooked with Garlic)

Serves 4

Ingredients

200g/7oz yoghurt

2 tbsp garlic paste

1 tsp garam masala

2 tbsp lemon juice

1 tsp ground black pepper

5 saffron strands

Salt to taste

750g/1lb 10oz boneless chicken, chopped into 8 pieces

2 tbsp refined vegetable oil

60ml/2fl oz double cream

Method

- Mix together the yoghurt, garlic paste, garam masala, lemon juice, pepper, saffron, salt and chicken. Refrigerate the mixture overnight.

- Heat the oil in a saucepan. Add the chicken mixture, cover with a lid and cook on a low heat for 40 minutes, stirring occasionally.

- Add the cream and stir for a minute. Serve hot.

Chicken Cafreal

(Goan Chicken in a Coriander Sauce)

Serves 4

Ingredients

1kg/2¼lb chicken, chopped into 8 pieces

5 tbsp refined vegetable oil

250ml/8fl oz water

Salt to taste

4 lemons, quartered

For the marinade:

50g/1¾oz coriander leaves, chopped

2.5cm/1in root ginger

10 garlic cloves

120ml/4fl oz malt vinegar

1 tbsp garam masala

Method

- Mix all the marinade ingredients together and grind with enough water to form a smooth paste. Marinate the chicken with this mixture for an hour.
- Heat the oil in a saucepan. Add the marinated chicken and fry on a medium heat for 5 minutes. Add the water and salt. Cover with a lid and simmer for 40 minutes, stirring occasionally. Serve hot with the lemons.

Chicken with Apricots

Serves 4

Ingredients

4 tbsp refined vegetable oil

3 large onions, finely sliced

1 tsp ginger paste

1 tsp garlic paste

1kg/2¼lb chicken, chopped into 8 pieces

1 tsp chilli powder

1 tsp turmeric

2 tsp ground cumin

2 tbsp sugar

300g/10oz dried apricots, soaked for 10 minutes

60ml/2fl oz water

1 tbsp malt vinegar

Salt to taste

Method

- Heat the oil in a saucepan. Add the onions, ginger paste and garlic paste. Fry on a medium heat till the onions are brown.

- Add the chicken, chilli powder, turmeric, ground cumin and sugar. Mix well and fry for 5-6 minutes.

- Add the remaining ingredients. Simmer for 40 minutes and serve hot.

Grilled Chicken

Serves 4

Ingredients

Salt to taste

1 tbsp malt vinegar

1 tsp ground black pepper

1 tsp ginger paste

1 tsp garlic paste

2 tsp garam masala

1kg/2¼lb chicken, chopped into 8 pieces

2 tbsp ghee

2 large onions, sliced

2 tomatoes, finely chopped

Method

- Mix the salt, vinegar, pepper, ginger paste, garlic paste and garam masala together. Marinate the chicken with this mixture for an hour.
- Heat the ghee in a saucepan. Add the onions and fry on a medium heat till they turn brown.
- Add the tomatoes and marinated chicken. Mix thoroughly and fry for 4-5 minutes.
- Remove from the heat and grill the mixture for 40 minutes. Serve hot.

Pepper Duck Roast

Serves 4

Ingredients

2 tbsp malt vinegar

1½ tsp ginger paste

1 tsp garlic paste

Salt to taste

1 tsp ground black pepper

1kg/2¼lb duck

2 tbsp butter

2 tbsp refined vegetable oil

3 large onions, finely sliced

4 tomatoes, finely chopped

1 tsp sugar

500ml/16fl oz water

Method

- Mix the vinegar, ginger paste, garlic paste, salt and pepper. Pierce the duck with a fork and marinate with this mixture for 1 hour.
- Heat the butter and oil together in a saucepan. Add the onions and tomatoes. Fry on a medium heat for 3-4 minutes. Add the duck, sugar and water. Mix well and simmer for 45 minutes. Serve hot.

Bhuna Chicken

(Chicken cooked in Yoghurt)

Serves 4

Ingredients

4 tbsp refined vegetable oil

1kg/2¼lb chicken, chopped into 12 pieces

1 tsp ginger paste

1 tsp garlic paste

½ tsp turmeric

2 large onions, finely chopped

1½ tsp garam masala

1 tsp freshly ground black pepper

150g/5½oz yoghurt, whisked

Salt to taste

Method

- Heat the oil in a saucepan. Add the chicken and fry on a medium heat for 6-7 minutes. Drain and set aside.
- To the same oil, add the ginger paste, garlic paste, turmeric and onions. Fry on a medium heat for 2 minutes, stirring frequently.
- Add the fried chicken and all the remaining ingredients. Cook for 40 minutes on a low heat. Serve hot.

Chicken Curry with Eggs

Serves 4

Ingredients

6 garlic cloves

2.5cm/1in root ginger

25g/scant 1oz grated fresh coconut

2 tsp poppy seeds

1 tsp garam masala

1 tsp cumin seeds

1 tbsp coriander seeds

1 tsp turmeric

Salt to taste

4 tbsp refined vegetable oil

2 large onions, finely chopped

1kg/2¼lb chicken, chopped into 8 pieces

4 eggs, hard-boiled and halved

Method

- Grind together the garlic, ginger, coconut, poppy seeds, garam masala, cumin seeds, coriander seeds, turmeric and salt. Set aside.

- Heat the oil in a saucepan. Add the onions and the ground paste. Fry on a medium heat for 3-4 minutes. Add the chicken and mix well to coat.

- Simmer for 40 minutes. Garnish with the eggs and serve hot.

Chicken Fried with Spices

Serves 4

Ingredients

1kg/2¼lb chicken, chopped into 8 pieces

250ml/8fl oz refined vegetable oil

For the marinade:

1½ tsp ground coriander

4 green cardamom pods

7.5cm/3in cinnamon

½ tsp fennel seeds

1 tbsp garam masala

4-6 garlic cloves

2.5cm/1in root ginger

1 large onion, grated

1 large tomato, puréed

Salt to taste

Method

- Grind all the marinade ingredients together. Marinate the chicken with this mixture for 30 minutes.
- Cook the marinated chicken in a saucepan on a medium heat for 30 minutes, stirring occasionally.
- Heat the oil and fry the cooked chicken for 5-6 minutes. Serve hot.

Goan Kombdi

(Goan Chicken Curry)

Serves 4

Ingredients

1kg/2¼lb chicken, chopped into 8 pieces

Salt to taste

½ tsp turmeric

6 red chillies

5 cloves

5cm/2in cinnamon

1 tbsp coriander seeds

½ tsp fenugreek seeds

½ tsp mustard seeds

4 tbsp oil

1 tbsp tamarind paste

500ml/16fl oz coconut milk

Method

- Marinate the chicken with the salt and turmeric for 1 hour. Set aside.
- Grind together the chillies, cloves, cinnamon, coriander seeds, fenugreek seeds and mustard seeds with enough water to form a paste.
- Heat the oil in a saucepan. Fry the paste for 4 minutes. Add the chicken, tamarind paste and coconut milk. Simmer for 40 minutes and serve hot.

South Chicken Curry

Serves 4

Ingredients

16 cashew nuts

6 red chillies

2 tbsp coriander seeds

½ tsp cumin seeds

1 tbsp lemon juice

5 tbsp ghee

3 large onions, finely chopped

10 garlic cloves, finely chopped

2.5cm/1in root ginger, finely chopped

1kg/2¼lb chicken, chopped into 12 pieces

1 tsp turmeric

Salt to taste

500ml/16fl oz coconut milk

Method

- Grind the cashew nuts, red chillies, coriander seeds, cumin seeds and lemon juice with enough water to form a smooth paste. Set aside.
- Heat the ghee. Add the onions, garlic and ginger. Fry for 2 minutes.
- Add the chicken, turmeric, salt and the cashew nut paste. Fry for 5 minutes. Add the coconut milk and simmer for 40 minutes. Serve hot.

Nizami Chicken

(Chicken cooked with Saffron and Almonds)

Serves 4

Ingredients

4 tbsp refined vegetable oil

1 large chicken, chopped into 8 pieces

Salt to taste

750ml/1¼ pints milk

½ tsp saffron, soaked in 2 tsp milk

For the spice mixture:

1 tbsp ginger paste

3 tbsp poppy seeds

5 red chillies

25g/scant 1oz desiccated coconut

20 almonds

6 tbsp milk

Method

- Grind the spice mixture ingredients together to form a smooth paste.

- Heat the oil in a saucepan. Fry the paste on a low heat for 4 minutes.

- Add the chicken, salt and milk. Simmer for 40 minutes, stirring frequently. Add the saffron and simmer for another 5 minutes. Serve hot.

Duck Buffad

(Duck cooked with Vegetables)

Serves 4

Ingredients

4 tbsp ghee

3 large onions, quartered

750g/1lb 10oz duck, chopped into 8 pieces

3 large potatoes, quartered

50g/1¾oz cabbage, chopped

200g/7oz frozen peas

1 tsp turmeric

4 green chillies, slit lengthways

1 tsp ground cinnamon

1 tsp ground cloves

30g/1oz mint leaves, finely chopped

Salt to taste

750ml/1¼ pints water

1 tbsp malt vinegar

Method

- Heat the ghee in a saucepan. Add the onions and fry on a medium heat till brown. Add the duck and sauté for 5-6 minutes.
- Add the remaining ingredients, except the water and vinegar. Fry for 8 minutes. Add the water and vinegar. Simmer for 40 minutes. Serve hot.

Adraki Murgh

(Ginger Chicken)

Serves 4

Ingredients

2 tbsp refined vegetable oil

2 large onions, finely chopped

2 tbsp ginger paste

½ tsp garlic paste

½ tsp turmeric

1 tbsp garam masala

1 tomato, finely chopped

1kg/2¼lb chicken, chopped into 12 pieces

Salt to taste

Method

- Heat the oil in a saucepan. Add the onions, ginger paste and garlic paste and fry on a medium heat for 1-2 minutes.
- Add all the remaining ingredients and sauté for 5-6 minutes.
- Grill the mixture for 40 minutes and serve hot.

Bharva Murgh

(Stuffed Chicken)

Serves 4

Ingredients

½ tsp ginger paste

½ tsp garlic paste

1 tsp tamarind paste

1kg/2¼lb chicken

75g/2½oz ghee

2 large onions, finely chopped

Salt to taste

3 large potatoes, chopped

2 tsp ground coriander

1 tsp ground cumin

1 tsp mustard powder

50g/1¾oz coriander leaves, chopped

2 cloves

2.5cm/1in cinnamon

Method

- Mix the ginger, garlic and tamarind pastes. Marinate the chicken with the mixture for 3 hours. Set aside.
- Heat the ghee in a saucepan and fry the onions till brown. Add all the remaining ingredients, except the marinated chicken. Fry for 6 minutes.
- Stuff this mixture into the marinated chicken. Roast in an oven at 190°C (375°F, Gas Mark 5) for 45 minutes. Serve hot.

Malaidar Murgh

(Chicken cooked in Creamy Gravy)

Serves 4

Ingredients

4 tbsp refined vegetable oil

2 large onions, finely chopped

¼ tsp ground cloves

Salt to taste

1kg/2¼lb chicken, chopped into 12 pieces

250ml/8fl oz water

3 tomatoes, finely chopped

125g/4½oz yoghurt, whisked

500ml/16fl oz single cream

2 tbsp cashew nuts, ground

10g/¼oz coriander leaves, chopped

Method

- Heat the oil in a saucepan. Add the onions, cloves and salt. Fry on a medium heat for 3 minutes. Add the chicken and sauté for 7-8 minutes.

- Add the water and tomatoes. Cook for 30 minutes.

- Add the yoghurt, cream and cashew nuts. Simmer for 10 minutes.

- Garnish with the coriander leaves and serve hot.

Bombay Chicken Curry

Serves 4

Ingredients

8 tbsp refined vegetable oil

1kg/2¼lb chicken, chopped into 12 pieces

2 large onions, sliced

1 tsp ginger paste

1 tsp garlic paste

4 cloves, ground

2.5cm/1in cinnamon, ground

1 tsp ground cumin

Salt to taste

2 tomatoes, finely chopped

500ml/16fl oz water

Method

- Heat half the oil in a frying pan. Add the chicken and fry on a medium heat for 5-6 minutes. Set aside.

- Heat the remaining oil in a saucepan. Add the onions, ginger paste and garlic paste and fry on a medium heat till the onions turn brown. Add the remaining ingredients, except the water and chicken. Sauté for 5-6 minutes.

- Add the fried chicken and water. Simmer for 30 minutes and serve hot.

Durbari Chicken

(Rich Gravy Chicken)

Serves 4

Ingredients

150g/5½oz chana dhal*

Salt to taste

1 litre/1¾ pints water

2.5cm/1in root ginger

10 garlic cloves

4 red chillies

3 tbsp ghee

2 large onions, finely chopped

½ tsp turmeric

2 tbsp garam masala

½ tbsp poppy seeds

2 tomatoes, finely chopped

1kg/2¼lb chicken, chopped into 10-12 pieces

2 tsp tamarind paste

20 cashew nuts, ground to a paste

250ml/8fl oz water

250ml/8fl oz coconut milk

Method

- Mix the dhal with salt and half the water. Cook in a saucepan on a medium heat for 45 minutes. Grind to a paste with the ginger, garlic and red chillies.
- Heat the ghee in a saucepan. Add the onions, dhal mixture and turmeric. Fry on a medium heat for 3-4 minutes. Add all the remaining ingredients.
- Mix well and simmer for 40 minutes, stirring occasionally. Serve hot.

Duck Fry

Ingredients

3 tbsp malt vinegar

2 tbsp ground coriander

½ tsp ground black pepper

Salt to taste

1kg/2¼lb duck, chopped into 8 pieces

60ml/2fl oz refined vegetable oil

2 small onions

1 litre/1¾ pints hot water

Method

- Mix the vinegar with the ground coriander, pepper and salt. Marinate the duck with this mixture for 1 hour.
- Heat the oil in a saucepan. Fry the onions on a medium heat till brown.
- Add the water, salt and the duck. Simmer for 45 minutes and serve hot.

Coriander Garlic Chicken

Serves 4

Ingredients

4 tbsp refined vegetable oil

5cm/2in cinnamon

3 green cardamom pods

4 cloves

2 bay leaves

3 large onions, finely chopped

10 garlic cloves, finely chopped

1 tsp ginger paste

3 tomatoes, finely chopped

1 large chicken, chopped

250ml/8fl oz water

150g/5½oz coriander leaves, chopped

Salt to taste

Method

- Heat the oil in a saucepan. Add the cinnamon, cardamom, cloves, bay leaves, onions, garlic and ginger paste. Fry for 2-3 minutes.
- Add all the remaining ingredients. Simmer for 40 minutes and serve hot.

Masala Duck

Serves 4

Ingredients

30g/1oz ghee plus 1 tbsp for frying

1 large onion, finely sliced

1 tsp ginger paste

1 tsp garlic paste

1 tsp ground coriander

½ tsp ground black pepper

1 tsp turmeric

1kg/2¼lb duck, chopped into 12 pieces

1 tbsp malt vinegar

Salt to taste

5cm/2in cinnamon

3 cloves

1 tsp mustard seeds

Method

- Heat 30g/1oz of the ghee in a saucepan. Add the onion, ginger paste, garlic paste, coriander, pepper and turmeric. Fry for 6 minutes.

- Add the duck. Fry on a medium heat for 5 minutes. Add the vinegar and salt. Mix well and simmer for 40 minutes. Set aside.

- Heat the remaining ghee in a saucepan and add the cinnamon, cloves and mustard seeds. Let them splutter for 15 seconds. Pour this over the duck mixture and serve hot.

Mustard Chicken

Serves 4

Ingredients

2 large tomatoes, finely chopped

10g/¼oz mint leaves, finely chopped

30g/1oz coriander leaves, chopped

2.5cm/1in root ginger, peeled

8 garlic cloves

3 tbsp mustard oil

2 tsp mustard seeds

½ tsp fenugreek seeds

1kg/2¼lb chicken, chopped into 12 pieces

500ml/16fl oz warm water

Salt to taste

Method

- Grind the tomatoes, mint leaves, coriander leaves, ginger and garlic to a smooth paste. Set aside.
- Heat the oil in a saucepan. Add the mustard seeds and fenugreek seeds. Let them splutter for 15 seconds.
- Add the tomato paste and fry on a medium heat for 2-3 minutes. Add the chicken, water and salt. Mix well and simmer for 40 minutes. Serve hot.

Murgh Lassanwallah

(Garlic Chicken)

Serves 4

Ingredients

400g/14oz yoghurt

3 tsp garlic paste

1½ tsp garam masala

Salt to taste

750g/1lb 10oz boneless chicken, chopped into 12 pieces

1 tbsp refined vegetable oil

1 tsp cumin seeds

25g/scant 1oz dill leaves

500ml/16fl oz milk

1 tbsp ground black pepper

Method

- Mix the yoghurt, garlic paste, garam masala and salt together. Marinate the chicken with this mixture for 10-12 hours.

- Heat the oil. Add the cumin seeds and let them splutter for 15 seconds. Add the marinated chicken and fry on a medium heat for 20 minutes.

- Add the dill leaves, milk and pepper. Simmer for 15 minutes. Serve hot.

Pepper Chicken Chettinad

(South Indian Pepper Chicken)

Serves 4

Ingredients

2½ tbsp refined vegetable oil

10 curry leaves

3 large onions, finely chopped

1 tsp ginger paste

1 tsp garlic paste

½ tsp turmeric

2 tomatoes, finely chopped

½ tsp ground fennel seeds

¼ tsp ground cloves

500ml/16fl oz water

1kg/2¼lb chicken, chopped into 12 pieces

Salt to taste

1½ tsp coarsely ground black pepper

Method

- Heat the oil in a saucepan. Add the curry leaves, onions, ginger paste and garlic paste. Fry on a medium heat for a minute.

- Add all the remaining ingredients. Simmer for 40 minutes and serve hot.

Chicken Mince with Eggs

Serves 4

Ingredients

3 tbsp refined vegetable oil

4 eggs, hard-boiled and sliced

2 large onions, finely chopped

2 tsp ginger paste

2 tsp garlic paste

2 tomatoes, finely chopped

1 tsp ground cumin

2 tsp ground coriander

½ tsp turmeric

8-10 curry leaves

1 tsp garam masala

750g/1lb 10oz chicken, minced

Salt to taste

360ml/12fl oz water

Method

- Heat the oil in a saucepan. Add the eggs. Fry for 2 minutes and set aside.
- To the same oil, add the onions, ginger paste and garlic paste. Fry on a medium heat for 2-3 minutes.
- Add all the remaining ingredients, except the water. Mix well and fry for 5 minutes. Add the water. Simmer for 30 minutes.
- Garnish with the eggs. Serve hot.

Dry Chicken

Serves 4

Ingredients

1kg/2¼lb chicken, chopped into 12 pieces

6 tbsp refined vegetable oil

3 large onions, thinly sliced

For the marinade:

8 red chillies

1 tbsp sesame seeds

1 tbsp coriander seeds

1 tsp garam masala

4 green cardamom pods

10 garlic cloves

3.5cm/1½in root ginger

6 tbsp malt vinegar

Salt to taste

Method

- Grind all the marinade ingredients together to a smooth paste. Marinate the chicken with this paste for 3 hours.

- Heat the oil in a saucepan. Fry the onions on a low heat till brown. Add the chicken and cook for 40 minutes, stirring frequently. Serve hot.

Prawn Curry Rosachi

(Prawns cooked with Coconut)

Serves 4

Ingredients

200g/7oz fresh coconut, grated

5 red chillies

1½ tsp coriander seeds

1½ tsp poppy seeds

1 tsp cumin seeds

½ tsp turmeric

6 garlic cloves

120ml/4fl oz refined vegetable oil

2 large onions, finely chopped

2 tomatoes, finely chopped

250g/9oz prawns, shelled and de-veined

Salt to taste

Method

- Grind the coconut, red chillies, coriander, poppy seeds, cumin seeds, turmeric and garlic with enough water to form a smooth paste. Set aside.

- Heat the oil in a saucepan. Fry the onions on a low heat till brown.

- Add the ground coconut-red chillies paste, tomatoes, prawns and salt. Mix well. Cook for 15 minutes, stirring occasionally. Serve hot.

Fish Stuffed with Dates & Almonds

Serves 4

Ingredients

4 trout, 250g/9oz each, slit vertically

½ tsp chilli powder

1 tsp ginger paste

250g/9oz fresh seedless dates, blanched and finely chopped

75g/2½oz almonds, blanched and finely chopped

2-3 tbsp steamed rice (see here)

1 tsp sugar

¼ tsp ground cinnamon

½ tsp ground black pepper

Salt to taste

1 large onion, finely sliced

Method

- Marinate the fish with the chilli powder and ginger paste for 1 hour.

- Mix the dates, almonds, rice, sugar, cinnamon, pepper and salt together. Knead to form a soft dough. Set aside.

- Stuff the date-almond dough in the slits of the marinated fish. Place the stuffed fish on a sheet of aluminium foil and sprinkle the onion on top.

- Wrap the fish and onion inside the foil and seal the edges firmly.

- Bake in an oven at 200°C (400°F, Gas Mark 6) for 15-20 minutes. Unwrap the foil and bake the fish for 5 more minutes. Serve hot.

Tandoori Fish

Serves 4

Ingredients

1 tsp ginger paste

1 tsp garlic paste

½ tsp garam masala

1 tsp chilli powder

1 tbsp lemon juice

Salt to taste

500g/1lb 2oz monkfish tail fillets

1 tbsp chaat masala*

Method

- Mix together the ginger paste, garlic paste, garam masala, chilli powder, lemon juice and salt.

- Make incisions on the fish. Marinate with the ginger-garlic mixture for 2 hours.

- Grill the fish for 15 minutes. Sprinkle with the chaat masala. Serve hot.

Fish with Vegetables

Serves 4

Ingredients

750g/1lb 10oz salmon fillets, skinned

½ tsp turmeric

Salt to taste

2 tbsp mustard oil

¼ tsp mustard seeds

¼ tsp fennel seeds

¼ tsp onion seeds

¼ tsp fenugreek seeds

¼ tsp cumin seeds

2 bay leaves

2 dry red chillies, halved

1 large onion, finely sliced

2 large green chillies, slit lengthways

½ tsp sugar

125g/4½oz canned peas

1 large potato, chopped into strips

2-3 small aubergines, julienned

250ml/8fl oz water

Method

- Marinate the fish with the turmeric and salt for 30 minutes.

- Heat the oil in a saucepan. Add the marinated fish and fry on a medium heat for 4-5 minutes, turning occasionally. Drain and set aside.

- To the same oil, add the mustard, fennel, onion, fenugreek and cumin seeds. Let them splutter for 15 seconds.

- Add the bay leaves and red chillies. Fry for 30 seconds.

- Add the onion and green chillies. Fry on a medium heat till the onion turns brown.

- Add the sugar, peas, potato and aubergines. Mix well. Stir-fry the mixture for 7-8 minutes.

- Add the fried fish and the water. Mix well. Cover with a lid and simmer for 12-15 minutes, stirring occasionally.

- Serve hot.

Tandoor Gulnar

(Trout cooked in a Tandoor)

Serves 4

Ingredients

4 trout, 250g/9oz each

Butter for basting

For the first marinade:

120ml/4fl oz malt vinegar

2 tbsp lemon juice

2 tsp garlic paste

½ tsp chilli powder

Salt to taste

For the second marinade:

400g/14oz yoghurt

1 egg

1 tsp garlic paste

2 tsp ginger paste

120ml/4fl oz fresh single cream

180g/6½oz besan*

Prawns in Green Masala

Serves 4

Ingredients

1cm/½in root ginger

8 garlic cloves

3 green chillies, slit lengthways

50g/1¾oz coriander leaves, chopped

1½ tbsp refined vegetable oil

2 large onions, finely chopped

2 tomatoes, finely chopped

500g/1lb 2oz large prawns, shelled and de-veined

1 tsp tamarind paste

Salt to taste

½ tsp turmeric

Method

- Grind together the ginger, garlic, chillies and coriander leaves. Set aside.
- Heat the oil in a saucepan. Fry the onions on a low heat till brown.
- Add the ginger-garlic paste and the tomatoes. Fry for 4-5 minutes.
- Add the prawns, tamarind paste, salt and turmeric. Mix well. Cook for 15 minutes, stirring occasionally. Serve hot.

Fish Cutlet

Serves 4

Ingredients

2 eggs

1 tbsp plain white flour

Salt to taste

400g/14oz John Dory, skinned and filleted

500ml/16fl oz water

2 large potatoes, boiled and mashed

1½ tsp garam masala

1 large onion, grated

1 tsp ginger paste

Refined vegetable oil for deep frying

200g/7oz breadcrumbs

Method

- Whisk the eggs with the flour and salt. Set aside.
- Cook the fish in salted water in a saucepan on a medium heat for 15-20 minutes. Drain and knead with the potatoes, garam masala, onion, ginger paste and salt to a soft dough.
- Divide into 16 portions, roll into balls and flatten lightly to form cutlets.
- Heat the oil in a pan. Dip the cutlets in the whisked egg, roll in the breadcrumbs and deep fry on a low heat till golden brown. Serve hot.

Parsi Fish Sas

(Fish cooked in White Sauce)

Serves 4

Ingredients

1 tbsp rice flour

1 tbsp sugar

60ml/2fl oz malt vinegar

2 tbsp refined vegetable oil

2 large onions, finely sliced

½ tsp ginger paste

½ tsp garlic paste

1 tsp ground cumin

Salt to taste

250ml/8fl oz water

8 fillets lemon sole

2 eggs, whisked

Method

- Grind the rice flour with the sugar and vinegar to a paste. Set aside.
- Heat the oil in a saucepan. Fry the onions on a low heat till brown.
- Add the ginger paste, garlic paste, ground cumin, salt, water and fish. Cook on a low heat for 25 minutes, stirring occasionally.
- Add the flour mixture and cook for a minute.
- Gently add the eggs. Stir for a minute. Garnish and serve hot.

Peshawari Machhi

Ingredients

3 tbsp refined vegetable oil

1kg/2¼lb salmon, sliced into steaks

2.5cm/1in root ginger, grated

8 garlic cloves, crushed

2 large onions, ground

3 tomatoes, blanched and chopped

1 tsp garam masala

400g/14oz yoghurt

¾ tsp turmeric

1 tsp amchoor*

Salt to taste

Method

- Heat the oil. Fry the fish on a low heat till golden. Drain and set aside.
- To the same oil, add the ginger, garlic and onions. Fry on a low heat for 6 minutes. Add the fried fish and all the remaining ingredients. Mix well.
- Simmer for 20 minutes and serve hot.

Crab Curry

Serves 4

Ingredients

4 medium-sized crabs, cleaned (see <u>cooking techniques</u>)

Salt to taste

1 tsp turmeric

½ coconut, grated

6 garlic cloves

4-5 red chillies

1 tbsp coriander seeds

1 tbsp cumin seeds

1 tsp tamarind paste

3-4 green chillies, slit lengthways

1 tbsp refined vegetable oil

1 large onion, finely chopped

Method

- Marinate the crabs with the salt and turmeric for 30 minutes.
- Grind all the remaining ingredients, except the oil and onion, with enough water to form a smooth paste.
- Heat the oil in a saucepan. Fry the ground paste and the onion on a low heat till the onion are brown. Add some water. Simmer for 7-8 minutes, stirring occasionally. Add the marinated crabs. Mix well and simmer for 5 minutes. Serve hot.

Mustard Fish

Serves 4

Ingredients

8 tbsp mustard oil

4 trout, 250g/9oz each

2 tsp ground cumin

2 tsp ground mustard

1 tsp ground coriander

½ tsp turmeric

120ml/4fl oz water

Salt to taste

Method

- Heat the oil in a saucepan. Add the fish and fry it on a medium heat for 1-2 minutes. Flip the fish and repeat. Drain and set aside.
- To the same oil, add the ground cumin, mustard and coriander. Let them splutter for 15 seconds.
- Add the turmeric, water, salt and the fried fish. Mix well and simmer for 10-12 minutes. Serve hot.

Meen Vattichathu

(Red Fish cooked with Spices)

Serves 4

Ingredients

600g/1lb 5oz swordfish, skinned and filleted

½ tsp turmeric

Salt to taste

3 tbsp refined vegetable oil

½ tsp mustard seeds

½ tsp fenugreek seeds

8 curry leaves

2 large onions, finely sliced

8 garlic cloves, finely chopped

5cm/2in ginger, finely sliced

6 kokum*

Method

- Marinate the fish with the turmeric and salt for 2 hours.
- Heat the oil in a saucepan. Add the mustard and fenugreek seeds. Let them splutter for 15 seconds. Add all the remaining ingredients and the marinated fish. Stir-fry on a low heat for 15 minutes. Serve hot.

Lightning Source UK Ltd.
Milton Keynes UK
UKHW020639270521
384471UK00010B/819